NEURODYNAMICS OF MIND

Strategy for Treatment of Mental Illness

By
Binie Ver Lipps, M. Sc. Ph. D.
Ophidia Products, Inc.
4509 Mimosa Dr.
Bellaire, Texas 77401, USA

RoseDogBooks
PITTSBURGH PENNSYLVANIA 15222

The contents of this work including, but not limited to, the accuracy of events, people, and places depicted; opinions expressed; permission to use previously published materials included; and any advice given or actions advocated are solely the responsibility of the author, who asumes all liability for said work and indemnifies the publisher against any claims stemming from publication of the work.

All Rights Reserved
Copyright © 2008 by Binie Ver Lipps, M. Sc. Ph. D.
No part of this book may be reproduced or transmitted
in any form or by any means, electronic or mechanical,
including photocopying, recording, or by any information
storage and retrieval system without permission in
writing from the author.

ISBN: 978-1-4349-9133-1
Library of Congress control Number: 2008925168
Printed in the United States of America

First Printing

For information or to order additional books, please write:
Dorrance Publishing Co., Inc.
701 Smithfield Street, Third Floor
Pittsburgh, Pennsylvania 15222
U.S.A.
1-800-788-7654

Or visit our website and online catalogue at
www.rosedogbookstore.com

The book is dedicated in loving memory of my physicist husband Frederick W. Lipps, Ph. D.

TABLE OF CONTENTS

Preface .... v-xiv

Chapter 1 Psychology does not Exist 1-5

Chapter 2. Three Categories of Life 6-8

Chapter 3. Creation of Human Race 9-11

Chapter 4 Neurological Disorders 12-18

Chapter 5 Human Brain 19-20

Chapter 6. Treatment for Mental Illness 21-30

Chapter 7. Research in Animals 31-34

Chapter 8. Treatment for Mental Illness 35-51

Chapter 9. References Cited 52-53

PREFACE

I believe very little in psychology or in psychiatry therefore, I had never paid any attention to, or had thoughts about psychotherapy. I always questioned myself how can a psychologist read other person's mind, on which psychotherapy is based. I am a scientist currently involved in discovering treatment for neurological disorders. One of our therapeutics, ADESH discovered by me at my company Ophidia Products Inc., is for the treatment of Alzheimer's disease (AD). I got interested in psychology because of my personal exposure for thirty three years to the person, my husband Frederick Lipps who emerged with erratic behavior. My husband was a loving caring person. All of a sudden he became a different person. His behavior and the acts caused me hurt and pain emotionally.

I was trying to find out why my husband should behave and act the way he did. I did lot of reading and talking to the professionals in the fields of psychology, neurology and neurobiology. Most importantly, I got to learn about my husband's past life story by talking to him. Psychologist often wants to talk about the victim's mother, who has observed the behavior and characters from the birth. Furthermore, psychiatrists insist on having numerous sessions, once or twice a week for a prolong period of time, for months or years. Just like I learned by talking to Fred my husband over and over for a period of almost a year. Soon I realized that such behavior is psychological, related to the brain and translated in mind, to behave irrationally.

My husband told me that he had sex rejection while he was in his prime youth. He was so frustrated with the rejection that he had to undergo oral psychotherapy, for six months, with his parents consent. These events he told me after thirty four (33) years of marriage. This assault of sex rejection during his youth must have caused adverse effect on some part of his brain, some neurons must have lost the activity, became un functional and probably died off.

Two years before his death, I suppose, due to the past sex rejection my husband developed life style of lying, denial, being hostile, self centered and all these were enhanced after him becoming impotent. He was also secretive about his past, which I did not care to know. Apparently he wanted to have amnesia over these events. I was blind folded and committed to my marriage. My marriage to Fred was a first sight love and we had fairly good one for a period of 33 years. Fred was, a brilliant intellectual caring husband. I was trying my best to handle our lives together. If I have to describe my husband in one sentence, Fred was a brilliant, intellectual, tall handsome man and a great lover. He was everything to me, friend, consultant, adviser on every respect.

Recently scientists have found that controlling and suppression of unwanted memories is associated with reduced hippocampus activation and impaired retention of those memories. Furthermore, sex based erratic behavior emerges due to diverse factors and in older men reaching the impotency. Fred lost his man-hood, he became impotent and physically lost the ability for sex. He thought that was the end, perhaps sex was an important part of his life. He started complaining about constipation. Most men I know of Fred's age have some kind of sickness. Some have heart problem therefore bi-pass surgery. Some have prostate cancer or other type of cancer, diabetes and the most common reflux disorder. Such men with different types of sickness concentrate on survival, their main focus becomes survival and sex becomes subsidiary. My husband never had major sickness until he reached seventy two years of age.

Apparently, it seems that on becoming impotent, which he considered as sickness rather than a normal physiological aging process. I was unable to convince him that impotency is a normal process and all men have to reach to that stage, similarly that all women have to reach the stage of menopause.

Fred's misbehavior started by vanishing for three days without a trace. I knew that he was going away, but would not tell where. Such thing had not happened in thirty three years. I said good bye and left thr house. He was angry and he did not leave telephone number. All these years if either of us were away we would call each other every night. This is the first time that I was not able to reach him. It was horrifying to me. I do not know till this day how I must have survived, but I did, by burring myself in the laboratory, performing experiments for long hours. I felt like not going home when Fred was not going to be there. On fourth day Fred came home and it was a happy union. I was so glad to see him. That night after a long time we had physical love. I felt that it is all the past and hoped for the better. However, later Fred saw a lawyer behind my back and paid $ 2,500 as a retainer' fees so that he could file for a divorce. When I came to know I was devastated and became furious for his action therefore after two days he cancelled it. I had to fight with the lawyer to return the money. Finally we received $ 1,000 back. What a waste of money.

Since then I realized that Fred was having mental sickness and there is no real treatment. He lost thinking ability, he was not able distinguish from right and wrong. I thought my marriage and life was all over and I will have to live with it. Soon after his physical sickness started. His constipation became a severe problem which led into the diagnosis of "so called cancer". I started coining the constipation with impotency. I believe that at this stage of his life the neurons responsible for expelling and for erection must have became inactive or even died.

At this stage I can compare my last two years of marriage to that of Elizabeth Graham's marriage. Her husband, the president of the

Washington Post, over the Watergate scandal got very frustrated and started behaving and acting irrationally to the extent that he divorced his wife Elizabeth who realized that it was due his mental sickness, therefore she took him back Similarly, I realized that Fred was suffering from mental illness. I tried to ignore his erratic behavior and concentrated on how to improve his physical condition. Later Graham's mental illness became out of hand and he killed himself. It is known that 20 % of such afflicted people commit suicide. I was terrified that it may happen to me. Our physicist friend was placed in the psychiatric hospital for mental illness who committed suicide. Mathematicians and physicists are prone to commit suicide. My husband was a theoretical physicist, from Johns Hopkins. He died at the age of 75 years and 5 months. We were married for thirty five years and one month.

I am a scientist and very much interested in and involved in research in neurobiology and neurological disorders such as Alzheimer' disease (AD), Parkinson's disease (PD) and Down syndrome (DS) including other neurological disorders. AD and PD are diagnosed in later part of the life by clinical symptoms. For DS due to the trisomy of chromosome 21, causing retarded development of the brain, is diagnosed before the birth. AD, PD and DS are indeed neurological disorders which can be diagnosed. However, the mental neurological disorders and they are many, currently, based on behavior can not be diagnosed by any test, because there is none/. Such mental behavior is called psychology. According to the book, " Out of its Mind" by Hobson and Leonard, it is an accepted fact that psychiatry is in crisis and its fall from grace has a lot to do with our currently disgraceful treatment for mental illness because there is no suitable one.

Psychotherapy has come to loose its way, because the emerged drugs have failed to cure mental illness, on the contrary produce side effects. Thus we have come to the conclusion that mental illness is a misbehavior and it is not psychological, therefore, psychotherapy becomes irrelevant. So called psychology-mental behavior is merging with neurobiology. Mental illness is neurodynamics of mind. The entire neurobiology of brain depends upon neuron chemicals which are neuro trophins.

Nerve growth factor (NGF) was the first discovered neuro trophic factor more than half century.. Since its discovery it was contemplated its use to treat neurological disorders. However its use did not in practice because of the (**Blood-brain barrier (BBB)**. Unlike all other organs BBB regulates substances entering the brain via the blood circulation system. This barrier is a unique defense system, which shuts out most toxins, bacteria and viruses which may be circulating in the blood, but allows the entry of necessary blood born molecules such as oxygen and glucose. The brain accounts for about 20 percent of the total oxygen consumption of the body; the energy associated with oxygen consumption comes from the utilization of glucose.

The prospects for reforming and reviving psychiatry are brighter, because, the public wants treatment for mental illness. Such treatment is now feasible if the gap between psychotherapy and biomedicine is bridged. In this book I have proposed treatment of ADESH for mental illness. Therapeutic ADESH was developed for the treatment of Alzheimer in particular and neurological disorders in general including mental illness . The treatment of ADESH is based upon the biochemistry of brain affected by some insults, leading to mental behavior which translates into erratic behavior. The proposed therapy is scientifically and morally acceptable. The understanding has come at the right time because the public patience is wearing out. The public wants the treatment simple, effective without side effects. Neuroscience is pretty much in the dark about the mind and it is likely to remain so. Neuroscience can come out of dark by bridging mind with behavior.

Nerve growth factor was the first discovered neuro trophic factor. The control of neuro peptides over brain functions has lead to several hypotheses assuming disturbances in central peptidergic systems to be implicated in pathogenesis of various psychopathologic and disturbed behavior. My invention of discovering

ADESH, an analogue of nerve growth factor (NGF) is a synthetic peptide consisting of ten amino acids, for the treatment of neurological disorders, such as AD and PD. Down syndrome is in-born neurological disorder. Synthetic ADESH is non toxic can be administered by injection or orally under the tongue. Nerve growth factor and other neurotrophic factors are large molecules resists the penetration to brain given either by injection or orally. To the contrary, synthetic ADESH being a small molecule crosses the blood-brain barrier (BBB) and reaches the brain.

AD and DS both are cognitive disorders and mental illness/psychological misbehavior is due to cognitive assaults. Therefore, I believe that ADESH should be advocated to treat mental illness. On recognizing that a person is undergoing depression due to some kind of assault, if such person is treated with ADESH will restore the affected neurons, to normal state. In case of my husband ADESH would have not been effective, because the length of the period over forty years, the affected neurons must have been dead.

The drug Viagra activates erection in men is due to the increase in blood pressure. In several men Viagra produced blood pressure excessively and has killed them by heart attack. Moreover, effect of Viagra is temporary. I believe that if ADESH was given to my husband soon after he started complaining, it would have helped to activate the failing neurons for the task of erection, so that overcoming his problem of constipation. However, realization of this aspect of ADESH came to me after his death. He died at the age of 75 years and 5 months. We were married for thirty five years and one month.

In animals ADESH has shown to arrest aging. My research has revealed that the lower concentration of nerve growth factor is found in AD, PD and DS patients. Patients with DS show low NGF level from early age where as AD and PD show decrease level of NGF in comparison to normal counterpart, after the manifestation of the disease.

Normal adults loose 0.2 % brain volume per year, whereas in patients with Alzheimer's disease the loss is greater. This is a clear indication that the death of neurons causing decrease level of neurotrophins may be manifesting the AD condition. As we age the population of neurons goes down decreasing the neurotrophin concentration. Thus, theoretically AD and aging can be controlled by Neurotrophin treatment.

ADESH is advocated for the treatment of:
1. Neurological Disorders
2. Psychological disorders, which are mental illness.
3. Arresting Aging

Immunoglobulin E (IgE): Human immunoglobulins are different types, such as IgG, IgA, IgM, IgD and IgE. IgG, IgA and IgM are protective immunoglobulins and the role of IgD may be implicated for food allergy. IgE is a minor component of the total immunoglobulin and is implicated in allergy, which in some cases manifests asthma. Normal people have 0.2 to 1.0 mg % of IgE. My research has revealed that elevated level of IgE is implicated in various disorders: **(1)** Diabetes, **(2)** Autoimmune diseases, **(3)** Allergy/Asthma, **(4)** Depression **(5)** Adverse side effects to the chemotherapy in cancer patients. **(5)**. Osteoporosis **(6)** Chronic pain **(7)** Chronic inflammation. Currently, allergy is implicated with loss of eye vision.

My research has proved that the elevated level of IgE is a culprit in manifesting numerous disorders. Therefore, it is imperative to have treatment to lower IgE level. By bringing the IgE level to normal the symptoms for allergy, asthma and mental disorders will be reduced. IgE level fluctuates according to the environment, therefore, continuous treatment is advocated, because the mast cells persist for a long period of time. In this book I am advocating the treatment of newly discovered LT-10 to lower IgE level. Once the IgE level is brought down and maintained to normal status previous drugs will work better, because elevated IgE interferes with chemical drugs which are currently practiced.

FDA approved Xolair, Genentech Corporation humanized monoclonal anti-IgE antibody for treatment of asthma for people over twelve years of age neutralizes IgE. LT-10 also neutralizes IgE. LT-10 has several advantages over mono anti-IgE. LT-10 is a synthetic peptide made of ten amino acids, It can be made in abundance at low cost, where as the production of mono anti-IgE is expensive. LT-10 can be given under the tongue. Mono anti-IgE must be given by injection only. Both LT-10 and mono anti-IgE neutralize the circulating IgE and lowers its concentration. Percentage of asthma in children is increasing and mono anti-IgE is restricted to people above 12 years of age. For LT-10 there is no age limit.

LT-10 treatment is advocated to lower IgE concentration:
Which is implicated in various disorders:
(1) Diabetes,
(2) Autoimmune diseases,
(3) Allergy/Asthma, allergy affecting eye vision
(4) Depression
(5) Osteoporosis
(6) Chronic pain
(7) Chronic inflammation.
(8) Adverse side effects to the chemotherapy in cancer patients.

I always wonder about the therapeutics which worked in the past for mental illness quit working now. I am convinced by my research that this is due the elevated levels of IgE. The above mentioned disorders are treatable with LT-10 by lowering IgE concentration. Once the IgE level is brought down and maintained to normal status previous drugs will work better, because elevated IgE interferes with chemical drugs which are currently practiced.

I have advocated ADESH for controlling aging and LT-10 for lowering IgE is the outcome of my research. Both are patented technologies having several publications and presentations. I have been taking ADESH for several years and I feel physically and mentally alert, with great stamina. I have been taking LT-10 for several years that maintains my IgE level to the normal status, bringing other proteins to normal state. I used to be allergic to insects bite, now I am not.

CHAPTER 1
PSYCHOLOGY DOES NOT EXIST

What is psychology? There is no mention of psychology in the Bible or Quran. However, in some people throughout the New Testament there are references to demons and unclean spirits, which caused by altered irrational behavior. But those stories are regarded as mere ancient superstitions. Nevertheless, it is known for centuries, that some individuals are born with good mind and others with bad, just like most people are born right handed and few left handed. The behaviors of people today are the same as they were in time of Jesus. The only difference is that such kind of irrational behavior is called by the modern society as psychology or psychiatry, which is coined to many different names like paranoia, schizophrenia, depression etc. are all mental illness.

Depression: It is not just sadness due to failed romance or death of a loved one or disappointment in career. To feel sad and grief over such incidents is perfectly healthy and normal. However, such sadness and grief extends to abnormal length of time, it crosses into realm of mental illness, is termed as depression. It affects personal happiness, economic productivity and human life. People with such prolong mental history become grossly impaired in judgment, they can not distinguish between good and bad, or right and wrong. It has been documented that such afflicted people have history of home-wrecking, job-wrecking power and 20% of them commit suicide.

The people are still the same today as in the Bible times. To some extent every person is a demon-possessed. We possess some tendency to act against the highest and best within us. When the tendency gets out of control the irrational behavior occurs. Robert Owen who had adopted the teaching of materialistic philosophy has said, " *that man's character is a product, on one hand, of heredity; on the other, of the environment of the individual during his lifetime, and especially during his period of development*". Therefore, church affiliation right from infancy plays a great role. It is much easier to build up your faith with others than by yourself. That is why we have organized church. For many, faith in God comes normally and naturally because of the training we received by our godly parents.

Ten commandments of the bible emphasize how we lead our lives. It is very important for little children to teach to obey few of the ten commandments from the early age. They must be made aware of the difference between truth and lies. I participated in one day symposium "Healing: the Quest for Wholeness In Psychotherapy and Faith". One of the speakers Rabbi Simka Weintraub psychotherapist, said in his hand outs, " I, and many therapists don't believe in God and don't pray. How can I presume to discuss God and prayer with my clients?" I thought it was strange. If we do not believe in God then how can we emphasize the value of ten commandments? At the same symposium Dr. Gaband from Baylor College of Medicine, after telling several stories said that "we do not understand how psychotherapy works". On that I asked "If you do not understand how psychotherapy works, then how can you keep on practicing it"?. I did not get answer for my question because there is no answer for it.

In the 18th century nobody worried about what psychology was doing, because there was no psychology. Freud in 1895 noticed that many of his patients consulted him for neurological symptoms had no signs of brain disease. He proposed and developed "scientific" psychology which did not last because too little was known about the brain. When we talk about psychology it always means a bad behavior and wrong acts. Good minded people show good behavior and perform good behavior. It is not due to good psychology because there is no good psychology. The term psychology is always connected with bad, adverse, abnormal behavior and wrong acts.

The Bible tells us that we humans can suffer for our parents sins, before we reach adulthood, then we are on own. The parents of saints are found to be virtuous, having high morals and they were law abiding people. The individuals born with bad mind if not nurtured during the period of development can remain bad minded and commit irrational acts and behavior throughout their lives. Such individuals are considered as psychologically inflicted ones, by the psychologists. I consider them as people born with bad neurodynamics of mind. Why some are born that way, nobody can answer it. Every individual is God's creation. God creates all sort of people. Some of them are genius some are mentally retarded, some are beautiful some are ugly, some are tall some are short. Then there are people born with genetic disorders such as Down syndrome (DS), Phenylketonuria (PKU) and mny more.

Dementia is a symptom based on logical diagnosis in which there is loss of intellectual functioning severe enough to interfere with occupational or social functioning (American Psychiatric Association, 1987). Psychological testing for dementia of individuals with mental retardation generally begins with IQ test. Depressed people tend to complain about their lives and exaggerate their failures; whereas individuals with Alzheimer's disease tend to internalize their complains and to cover up their symptoms. The clinical diagnosis of dementia is difficult to make because according to Katzman1981, there are about 50 different causes of dementia in normal adults, who are not afflicted with AD. This clearly shows that there is difference between neurological disease AD and mental illness, although, both are cognitive disorders.

Schizophrenic psychoses: In my opinion the manifestation of adverse mind is considered to be due to psychology, by civilized, advanced society as we currently live in. Recently, scientists have come to understand that Schizophrenic psychoses as a change in mind due to decreased concentration of neurotrophic factor/s, leading to imbalanced homeostasis in the nervous system (Thome et al. 1998). Neurotrophic factor hypothesis states that existing neurons compete with each other for supply of neurotrophic factors/s provided by the target tissue or organ. Some survive and some do not survive and die. The loss of neurotrophic factor/s may cause manifestation of Alzheimer's disease or schizophrenia and other cognitive disorders. There are tests available to diagnose AD, PD and DS. However, there are no tests to diagnose mental illness/ psychological misbehavior which is also cognitive one.

My research has revealed that level of nerve growth factor, one of the several known neurotrophic factors, is low in patients suffering from AD, PD and DS. Neurotrophic factors are high molecular weight proteins, resists the penetration to brain given either by injection or orally. On injecting such high molecular weight protein will not be penetrated to the brain due to blood-brain-barrier (BBB). Unlike all other organs BBB regulates substances entering the brain via the blood circulation system. This barrier is a unique defense system, which shuts out most toxins, bacteria and viruses which may be circulating in the blood, but allows the entry of necessary blood born molecules such as oxygen and glucose. Orally taken proteins will be fragmented in the gut before absorbed in the body. Furthermore, injected protein will make antibodies which will interfere with the homeostasis. Therefore, it is imperative to discover a small molecule having neurotrophic activity capable of crossing BBB.

Thus it was imperative to discover small molecules having neurotrophic activity to overcome the BBB. Hefti et al. in their review article stated," *Rather than administrating entire trophic factor molecule, it may be possible to use modified molecules or active fragments. The development of non peptide agonistic molecules for neurotrophic factors which pass BBB is theoretically possible, may prove to be a Herculean task"*. My research at Ophidia Products,

Inc. the Herculean task has overcome by discovering synthetic ADESH, an analog of NGF consisting of ten amino acids which crosses BBB.

Nerve growth factor (NGF) is the first discovered neurotrophic factor. My painstaking research has identified the active domain for the biological activity of cobra venom derived NGF. The active domain consisting of 10 amino acids, in synthetic version mimics the biological properties of the whole molecule of NGF consisting of 116 amino acids. The synthetic version of the active domain of NGF is named ADESH. It can be made in abundance, and being a small molecule overcomes the blood-brain barrier. It can be administered by injection or can be taken by orally under the tongue. ADESH is advocated for treatment of cognitive disorders.

Chapter-2
THREE CATEGORIES OF LIFE

1. Imaginative State: Mostly children tend to live in the imaginative state. They imagine about things which do not exist, e.g. a bogy man and Santa Clause. As they grow up they come out of this state by proper environment, before they enter teen age. Nurturing environment is most essential for child's mental development. Retarded development of frontal lobes of the brain is related to antisocial behavior. In Down Syndrome (DS) victim besides frontal lobes, hippocampus appears to be reduced 30 to 50 %. There is an experimental proven evidence that controlling and suppressing unwanted memories are associated with reduced hippocampus activation and impaired retention of those memories.

During the last decades evidence has accumulated that pituitary and hypothalamic hormones, in addition to their classical endocrine action, affect particular functions of the central nervous system as well. Subsequently, it has been shown that pituitary hormones and variety of other neuro-peptides are present in the brain in more or less distinct neuronal pathways (Khachaturian et al 1985). The control of neuro-peptides over brain functions has led to several hypotheses assuming disturbances in central peptidergic systems to be implicated in the pathogenesis of various psychological disorders and disturbed behavior.

2. Realistic State: Most adults live in the realistic state. They have realized that life is short, and everyone has to face the problems and difficulties in life. They know that they have to behave well, make living by truthful service. They are also aware that death is inevitable. Some people, especially from the developing countries, survival becomes the main focus of their life. They labor hard, earn their living sincerely and live life realistically. Fortunately, most of the people live in realistic state.

3. Heroic State: White caller people having advanced degrees from the universities develop an aptitude towards becoming somebody, because financially they are O. K and therefore, survival is not a problem for them. Some succeed but most fail. In my opinion every Nobel Laureates is a hero, they worked hard for the highest recognition for their achievement. Mother Teresa became a hero while living, for her service to the poor dying people in Calcutta, India. Individual saint is a hero because they lived highly moral lives, suffered for their faith while living. Therefore they were canonized after a long time, sometimes several centuries after their death.

Jesse Jones and Bill Gates became rich in money and some may consider them as hero. Jesse Jones had 6th grade education and Bill Gates is a college drop out. However, in my opinion they are not real heroic, because they undermine the ambition of youngsters for higher education, which is the thrust of civilization of our time. Their riches came out of shear luck. However, their philanthropic attitude has made them famous and perhaps hero. It is important for all to have ambition for heroic goal. Some may even get obsessed become passionate to achieve their goal.

Some people never come out of the imaginative state. They tend to lead immature life, imaginatively. Their behavior becomes childish, immature and irrational. Andrea Yates imagined that demon was to hurt her children. It is like a child thinking that bogy man is going to take away his toys so he wants to hide them. Andrea Yates acted similarly in order not let her children run away, she made them still by killing them. This is a most sever case of mental illness. However, people who can not live realistically tend to behave irrationally, because they are living in a imaginative state.

Chapter-3
CREATION OF HUMAN RACE

God has created all sorts of people: people with physical defects, people with genetic and mental defects. Physical defects are obviously visible. Genetic and mental defects are not necessarily visible. Nevertheless, advanced scientific research has enabled to diagnose genetic defects. For example Down syndrome (DS) is a genetic condition of trisomy of chromosome 21 being in triplicate. DS is diagnosed before birth by amniocyntesis for extra chromosome and by ultrasonic testing for development of the fetus. DS victims are irritable, non-cooperative and suffer permanent defects in physical and verbal performance. There are 35,000 DS victims in the US alone and their IQ remains below 60.

Metabolic defects occur in the individuals born with missing gene. The individuals with missing gene for caseinase, show inability to digest foods containing casein containing dairy products. Due to this disorder scientific research came up with non dairy products to satisfy such individuals and to lead a happy normal lives. Phenylketanuria (PKU) is a genetic disorder in which the individuals are born with missing enzyme to digest essential amino acid phenyl alanine. Special food devoid of phenyl alanine is available for such individuals, which makes their lives almost normal.

God has created people with good mind and some with bad mind, just like people with genetic and metabolic defects, similarly, color blind and left and right handed people. Individuals born with good mind behave properly having good morals, are designated as normal people. However individuals born with bad mind behave abnormally, perform irrational acts which some times can be criminal. Such people are designated as bad people. Why does God create people with bad mind? Nobody has answer for it. It is the same way why God creates individuals with DS and other in born genetic disorders. Nobody can question God.

All my life I have been troubled by the Bible story, that Judas, one of the apostles of Jesus betrayed him. Jesus must have chosen very carefully his apostles and he loved them dearly. Why then Judas did get his mind converted to betrayal? Is it in the fulfillment of prophecy? Prophecy was laid by God and converted Judas loyal mind to bad mind to betray his Master. Therefore, I believe that God can act whichever way. God allows us to suffer probably: To get His attention, To develop righteousness, To teach us to be obedient, To develop character, perseverance. We do not understand it and therefore it is a "mistry". Almighty God can do good and bad for anybody. God is in power of good and bad. Lord gave and the Lord has taken away (Job 1:20). Shall we receive good at the hand of God and shall we not receive evil? (Job 2:10). How can we avoid God's anger towards us? Only answer I have is, prayer and obey the commandments. We must practice humility and have complete dependence and trust in God.

We all must believe in the followings:
1. Life is precious
2. Life is full of problems
3. Life is short
4. Death is inevitable

Life is precious: We all have a precious gift of life and therefore, in gratitude we remain embedded to our parents. Everyone must be passionate to live life and not just survive. Life is only one time, there is no second chance. We must extend every possible way to have peaceful and happy life. Scientists are working hard to discover new effective therapeutics to treat different diseases. Most of the therapeutics may not cure the disease but can prolong the life span and improve the quality of life. Suicide and killing must be considered sinful and immoral.

Life is full of problems There is no living person who does not have problems. Everyone has to lead difficult road of life. For some people the problems may not be as severe as for the others. Problems are not created by one self only, but many times they are brought by others. We know that the innocent people are persecuted and even killed. Is there any way that we can avoid injustice? I think and with my whole heart I believe that we must put complete faith in God and ask his guidance in leading our lives. We must practice humility and have complete dependence and trust in God.

Life is short: Nobody knows how long one can live. Some people live for 100 years while some die before the age 50 years. Is 100 and 50 years of age is short lived for these individuals? Not arithmetically. If we just know how long we will live, it would be easy for planning our lives. No, we cannot have planned lives because life is a mistry. .

Death is inevitable: Death is inevitable it is going to come to each one of us. However nobody knows when, that is a mistry. Some lucky ones die in their sleep. Some die instantly by accident. Some suffer from short or long illness before death.

Chapter-4
NEUROLOGICAL DISORDERS

Before 1750, insanity tended to be considered as an all-or-none metaphysical state relating to the body in an abstract way. The mind was fully alienated and there was little machinery for accounting for partial insanities, in spite of the fact that such states have been suggested. Currently, after a century, scientist have come to recognize the mental illness like schizophrenia, mania and depression are not the results of voodoo spells or demonic possession but instead are physical disorders of the brain. Neurobiology came out of the Civil War, inspired by examination of war related head injuries. It went on taking care of all brain diseases not presenting psychiatric symptoms. There are no tests or markers to recognize strictly mental illness contrary to as in physical disorders such as Alzheimer's and Parkinson's diseases, arthritis, Down syndrome (DS) and diabetes. These physical disorders are recognized by symptoms. DS is a trisomy of chromosome 21 is recognized before the birth of the victim. Chromosome 21 is also implicated in Alzheimer's disease. Research focused on chromosome 21 and DS resulted in the genes on chromosome 21 that play an important role in depression.

Alzheimer's Disease: Alzheimer's disease (AD) was first described in1907 by Dr. Alois Alzheimer, a German psychiatrist, who discovered large numbers of unusual microscopic deposits in the brain of demented patient upon autopsy. These deposits are now called amyloid plaques and neurofibrillary tangles, are highly insoluble protein aggregates. They are formed in the brains of Alzheimer's patients in particular regions, including those involved in memory. Plaques alone can constitute a significant portion of the mass of certain brain structures in advanced cases of the disease. Such massive plaque deposition is likely to affect brain function severely, and the affected brain regions demonstrate significant loss of specific populations of neurons. The actual loss of neurons as well as the impaired function of the surviving neurons are likely be the key to neuro-pathological contributors to the dementia that characterizes Alzheimer's disease. It is now known that there is a genetic factor in Alzheimer's disease, but there are also other causative factors and the chain of causation involving the amyloid protein is still a subject of research.

At present Alzheimer's disease can be conclusively diagnosed only by a histological examination of the brain after biopsy or autopsy. As a result, diagnosis of patients suspected of having Alzheimer's disease is typically made through a process of elimination, by conducting neurological and psychiatric examinations, extensive laboratory tests and possibly a brain scan, in order to rule out other conditions, such as stroke, brain tumor or depression, with similar symptoms. Alzheimer's disease typically follows a predictable course of deterioration over eight years or more, with the earliest symptoms being impairment of short term memory. Gradually, memory loss increases, reasoning deteriorates and the individual becomes depressed, agitated, irritable and restless. In the final stages of the disease, patients become totally unable to care for themselves. Death is often due to pneumonia or other related to the deteriorated physical condition of the patient

Alzheimer's disease is a neurodegenerative brain disorder leading to progressive memory loss, dementia, many signs of Parkinsonism and finally death. Memory loss begins with the recent memory and progresses toward a complete loss of mental function which reduces the victim to a vegetative state. This disorder is associated with loss of basal forebrain cholinergic neurons and accumulations of amyloid plaque in the brain. Alzheimer's disease is associated with markedly impaired cerebral glucose metabolism as detected by reduced cortical desoxy glucose utilization by altered activities of glycolytic enzymes or by reduced densities of cortical glucose transporter subtype. Both, cause and cure are unknown and although considerable efforts have been made, no prevention and no substantial remedy or remission is in current medical practice.

Alzheimer's disease is the fourth leading cause of death in the United States, responsible for approximately 100,000 deaths annually. By current estimates, over 2.5 million people in the United States alone suffer from Alzheimer's disease. Currently, there are approximately 25 million people affected by AD worldwide. It is estimated that, with the steady growth of over 65 years of age population, by the year 2030 this number will be greater than 60 million. In 2000, an estimated $100 billion was spent in the United States alone on health care expenses and lost wages for AD patients and their caregivers. The prediction is that by the year 2030, $375 billion will be spent annually.

Currently, four drugs, all in the same class have been approved by the FDA for the treatment of AD patients. These four drugs, Tacrine, Donepezil, Rivastigmine and Galantamine, are all inhibitors of acetyl chlinesterase and increase the level of acetylcholine in the brain. Although, these drugs temporarily improve cognition, global function and ability to conduct general activities necessary for daily living in some patients, they do not influence the progression of the disease. These class of drugs can be useful for relieving cognitive symptoms in some patients they do not work at all in advanced cases of AD.

There are continuous efforts being made by the scientists to discover new drugs for the treatment of AD The Apolipoprotein E (apoE) has been identified as a powerful risk factor for AD. The human apoE gene located on chromosome 19 has three Epson alleles, e2, e3 and e4 coding for three proteins: apoE2, apoE3 and EpoE4. The product of apoE gene is a 299 amino acid protein,

(Mahley 1988). The biochemical and physiological studies have defined a major role for this protein in lipid metabolism. In the central nervous system, apoE is the major lipid carrier protein and is involved in brain development and regeneration after injury (Cedazo-Minguez 2001). ApoE plays a role in both peripheral nervous system (PNS) and central nervous system (CNS). Initially, apoE was thought to be synthesized primarily by astrocytes but not by neurons in the brain. However, subsequent studies have demonstrated that the central nervous system neurons also express apoE under diverse physiological and pathological conditions. The brain is second only to the liver in abundance of apoE mRNA (Elshourbagy et al. 1985).

Several experimental drugs have been tried for AD:

1. Potential use of estrogen-like drugs for the prevention of Alzheimer's disease was a failure.

2. Immunological approach for the treatment of AD. Actve immunization with synthetic Abeta (1-42) peptide reduces Abeta plaques in amyloid precursor protein in transgenic mice without detectable toxicity., but extension of this approach to AD patients induced a neuro inflamatory reaction.

3. The possible role of tissue-type olasminogen activator (tPA) and tPA blockers in the pathogenesis and treatment of AD, the results were not conclusive. It has been documented that the amyloid precursor protein (APP) and the microtubule-associated protein tau, both have important roles in neuro-plasticity and memory function. Insulin degrading enzyme (IDE) is a protease that degrades insulin and the beta-amyloid peptide implicated in AD. In controlled experiments on humans, insulin-mediated glucose clearance was slower in e4-negative than in e4-positive AD cases (Craft et al. 1999).

4. AIT-082 is the first compound made by the company Neotherapeutics that entered human clinical trials for neuro-degen-

erative diseases, by oral administration. However, its efficacy was found to be marginal, showing no difference between Alzheimer's diseases patients treated with AIT-082 and placebo.

Down Syndrome: Down syndrome is a genetic condition of trisomy of chromosome 21, which is in triplicate. DS is named after Dr. John Langdon Down, an English physician who first described the characteristics of DS in 1866. It was not until 1959 that Jerome Leieune and Patricia Jacobs independently first determined the cause to be trisomy of the 21st chromosome. The chromosome 21 is triplicate in 96% DS individuals. Among people with Down syndrome 3 to 4% of have Robertsonian Translocation, where the extra chromosome is attached with chromosome 14.

The production of excessive beta amyloid plaques and amyloid angeopathy in DS and AD is linked to gene on human chromosome 21 that codes for beta-amyloid (Delabar et al.1987). Because of this relationship between DS and AD , it has been assumed that knowledge about almost any aspect of one of these conditions will illuminate the other (Mann et al. 1984).

DS children are born with physical abnormality in development of Eustachian tubes causing frequent ear infections. Structural abnormalities connected with the inadequate development of the entire maxillary region are very characteristic feature of DS and responsible for many facial features associated with trisomy 21. Persons with DS have increased susceptibility to infection due to the immunoglobulin subclass deficiency. Overall, respiratory infections remain a major problem. In addition, people with DS are at particularly high risk for AD, progressive dementia disorder with characteristic clinical signs and brain pathology. DS victims are irritable, non-cooperative and suffer permanent defects in physical and verbal performance. The IQ of DS remains below 60.

A muscular seizure is a loss of control of the body by the brain. From 5 to 10 % DS children have seizure problems. Some children with DS have a constipation condition referred as Hirscprung disease. Some DS babies are born with heart defects, some with the associated illnesses such as epilepsy, hypothyroidism or celiac disease. Most individuals with DS have developmental disabilities, such as developmental delay, speech abnormalities, and degrees of cognitive dysfunction. Post mortem examination of DS brains revealed that they are smaller than that of normal people. Hippocampus appears to be reduced to 30 to 50 % (Crome 1972). Antisocial behavior of DS is attributed to smaller size of frontal lobe. There is no treatment for DS victims.

Dementia: Dementia is a symtomological diagnosis in which there is loss of intellectual functioning severe enough to interfere with occupational or social functioning (American Psychiatric Association, 1987). Psychological testing for dementia of individuals with mental retardation generally begins with IQ test. Depressed people tend to complain about their lives and exaggerate their failures, where as individuals with AD tend to externalize their complains and to cover up their symptoms. The clinical diagnosis of dementia is difficult to make in individuals with DS. According to (Katzman 1981) there are about 50 different causes of dementia in normal adults. Once dementia has been documented individuals over the age of 30 years, the type must be established, — i.e., whether the dementia is a reversible condition such as reactive depression, endocrine and vitamin deficiencies, and uncontrolled seizures, or irreversible condition such as AD, subacute sclerotic panencephalitis, Creutzfeld-Jacob disease, AIDS and Huntington chorea. AD occurs in more than 50 % of all cases of dementia that are associated with old age.

Hypochondria: Individuals with hypochondria are preoccupied with health matters and unrealistic fears of disease. They are convinced that they have symptoms of physical illness, but their complaints typically do not confirm to any coherent pattern and they usually have trouble giving a precise description of their symptom. Mental Imagination, leading to negative effect h

Schizophrenia: Schizophrenia is one of the recognized mental illness. Schizophrenia is based on exclusion of other mental disorders. Positive symptoms approximately of three-fourth of schizophrenics show such as auditory hallucinations, delusions or cognitive disturbances World Health Organization (WHO 1973) report. Many researchers have reported that schizophrenic patients perform significantly worse than controls on the Wisconsin Card Sorting Test (WCST), this neurological test thought to be sensitive to frontal lobe dysfunction (Beatty et al. 1993; Sullivan et al. 1993). Nearly 99 % of schizophrenic patients show structural brain abnormalities specifically, enlarged ventricles.

For decades scientists have tried to search for the differences between normal individuals and schizophrenics, in blood serum. There is no marker which can reveal the mental ills. No one study can claim to give definitive answers to the question of what represents the neuropathology of schizophrenia and for other mental illness. Schizophrenic brains have shown to be significantly lighter than normal match (Brown et al. 1986). There was associated nerve loss in certain regions of brain in the schizophrenia group (Benes et al). There is a strong evidence for a generalized defect of cortical development in the schizophrenia group (Akbarian et al. 1993). It is now established that structural neuro-pathology exists in substantial proportion of schizophrenia like syndrome may arise as a result of gross brain lesion acquired in adult life.

Chapter 5
HUMAN BRAIN

Parts of Brain and their Functions: Brain is the most complex organ of the body. Most organs are transplantable from donor to the suffering recipient to improve the quality of life of the later. Brain is an exception. The brain is compartmentalized with different regions of brain doing different tasks. There are many parts which comprise the brain, each part having its own function. The hippocampus of the brain deals mainly with memory. The amygdala deals with fear and anxiety likewise hypothalamus with sleep, hunger and sex drive.

Brain consists of different areas specialized for different functions. Stephan et al. (2003) revealed different regions for different tasks in two hemi spears of the brain. The regions such as for language areas, region for judgment, region for sensory areas and control areas. Lateralized cognitive processes and lateralized task control human brain.

A neuro hormone can be released from both neural and non-neural cells, and most important to the definition, travels in some circulation to act at a distant from release site. For example, dopamine is a certified neurotransmitter in the striatum, yet it is released from the hypothalamus and travels through the hypophysial-portal circulation to the pituitary, where it inhibits the release of pro-lactin. Most peptides with their multiple activities in the brain and gut are generally considered to be neuro modulators. Nerve cells can conduct bioelectric signals for long distances without any loss of original strength. They possess specific intercellular connections with other nerve cells and with innervated tissues such as muscles and glands. Nerve cells are heterogeneous with respect to both size and shape.

Nowadays, neural systems and certain psychiatrics disorders are known to be linked. Major advances in neurosciences have opened up new research possibilities which have increased our understanding of the relationship between cerebral processes and behavioral, cognitive and emotional disorders. Most nerve cells (neurons) depend on chemical transmitters to send messages across the synapses. A chemical transmitter released into the gap provides communication across the gap. However, the chemicals neuro modulators after receiving by the neurons modulates the pattern of activity. A nerve impulse which is electrical in nature, travels from the cell body of a neuron down to the axon. There is only one axon for each neuron. Axons have branches at their end called axonal endings.

It is a basic feature of human experience to feel good in the presence of others and feel distressed when left behind. Different parts of the brain play a role for such feeling. The anterior cingulated cortex (ACC) is more active during close to people (inclusion). Right ventral prefrontal cortex (RVPEC) was active during depression. In human mothers, the ACC is activated by the sound of infant's cries. The authors N. I. Eisenberger et al. concluded that social and physical pain share a common neuro anatomical basis.

Chapter-6
TREATMENT FOR MENTAL ILLNESS

Psychiatry has come to loose its way, because emerged drugs have failed to cure mental illness, on the contrary produce side effects. Ironically, the drugs have improved and have become more versatile to treat wide range of mental ills, including schizophrenia, manic depressive illness and many anxiety disorders, but are not effective and not free from side effects.

Now we have come to the conclusion that mental illness is a misbehavior and it is not psychological, therefore, psychotherapy becomes irrelevant. So called psychology-mental behavior is merging with neurobiology. Mental illness is neurodynamics of mind. The entire neurobiology of brain depends upon neuro chemicals which are neurotrophins. Nerve growth factor was the first discovered neurotrophic factor. The control of neuro peptides over brain functions has lead to several hypotheses assuming disturbances in central peptidergic systems to be implicated in pathogenesis of various psychopathologic and disturbed behavior.

The prospects for reforming and reviving psychiatry are brighter, because, the public wants treatment for mental illness. Such treatment is now feasible if the gap between psychotherapy and biomedicine is bridged. In this book I have proposed treatment of ADESH for mental illness. Therapeutic ADESH primarily, was developed for the treatment of Alzheimer's disease in particular and neurological disorders in general including mental illness. The treatment of ADESH is based upon the biochemistry of brain affected by some insults, leading to mental behavior that translates into erratic behavior. The proposed therapy is scientifically and morally acceptable. The understanding has come at the right time because the public patience is wearing out. The public wants the treatment simple effective without side effects. Neuroscience is pretty much in the dark about the mind and it is likely to remain so. Neuroscience can come out of dark by bridging mind with behavior.

Snake Venoms: Snake venom is a complex mixture of many substances as toxins, enzymes, growth factors, activators and inhibitors with wide spectrum of biological activities. For a long time, it was believed that snake venom proteins have potential for treatment of cancer, viral diseases, epilepsy and neurological disorders such as Alzheimer's and Parkinson's diseases. The research at Ophidia Products, Inc. has translated this belief into reality, by discovering several novel patented proteins for treatment of cancer, wound healing, neurological disorders, and infections caused by RNA and DNA viruses. All these protein therapeutics are large molecules having high molecular weight and their preparation would dependeded on the natural source, which is venoms from various species of snakes. Hard and complicated research each one of these protein therapeutics are converted to synthetic version, to overcome blood-brain barrier (BBB) especially for the treatment of neurological disorders, Lipps 2000 patented therapeutics.

Nerve Growth Factor: First neurotrophic factor nerve growth factor (NGF) was discovered more than half a century ago (Levi-Montalcini et al. 1954). NGF is a progenitor of a family of growth factors (Hamburger 1993). Since the discovery of NGF several neurotrophic factors have been discovered: neurotrophin-3, neurotrophin-4/5, ciliary neurotrophic factor (CNTF), brain derived neurotrophic factor (BDNF) and glial cell neurotrophic factor (GCNF). These neurotrophic factors are large protein molecules produced by neural cells to regulate nerve cell growth and survival.

NGF, BDNF, NT-3 and NT-4/5 share approximately 50 % amino acid sequence identity (Hallbrook 1991).

NGF is the prototypic neurotrophic factor, that defines the properties and functions of the class of growth factors. NGF regulates the functions of the differentiated neurons. NGF is synthesized at a considerable distance from the cell body by peripheral tissues or other neurons that are contacted by axons of the NGF-sensitive neurons. Once the retrograde flow of NGF is established it must continue for the life time of the neuron to develop and maintain the functional differentiated state of the neurons (Barde 1989).

NGF is an important endogenous protein and its presence is not restricted to neural cells. Presence of NGF is reported in organs other than brain (Lipps 2000). NGF has been isolated from various non-neural cells (Lipps 2001), and from different body fluids such as saliva, serum and urine (Lipps 2000).

The concentration of NGF varies under stress, infection and intoxication. Emotional stress induced by parachute jumping changes blood nerve growth factor levels (Aloe et al. 1994). Lipps (2001) reported the decreased levels of NGF in organs of mice as a consequence of sub-lethal injection of cobra venom. My research has revealed that lower levels of NGF were observed in Alzheimer's disease where the patients are usually old. Low level of NGF was also observed in young people with Down syndrome. Furthermore, Lipps (2002) observed that the concentration of NGF in various organs of mice is age and gender dependant. There was decline in concentration of NGF as the age of male and female mice advanced. The concentration of NGF was found to be consistently higher in the organs of male mice than the female siblings at all ages.

Neurotrophic factor hypothesis states that developing neurons compete with each other for a limited supply of neurotrophic factor/s provided by the target tissue. Successful competitors survive, unsuccessful ones die. Loss of neurotrophic factor/s may cause manifestation of Alzheimer's disease or schizophrenia. It has been documented that in humans, schizophrenia is a mental disorder sharply increases between ages 15 and 35 years and slowly declines. After the age of 55 only few cases of schizophrenia appear. This observation is now out dated.

According to the mal developmental hypothesis neurotrophins might be genetically and neuro-chemically involved in etio-pathogenesis of schizophrenia psychosis (Thome et al. 1998). Patients suffering from schizophrenia psychosis and control persons were pheno typed for a null mutation of the ciliary neurotrophic factor gene and found no difference (Thome et al.1997). Preliminary clinical studies indicate that schizophrenia psychosis may be associated with changes in the genetic code of certain neurotrophic factors (Jansson et al. 1997). Studies of brain anatomy and pre-morbid functioning indicate that schizophrenia psychosis and other mental ills may be neuro-developmental origin. It further supports for an association between NT-3 gene and certain forms of schizophrenia psychosis (Jansson et al. 1997).

Different types of insults can cause a change in the concentration of neurotrophins and imbalance in homeostasis, leading to schizophrenic psychosis and other mental ills. The insults can be as follows:

1. Physical trauma; accident, fall etc.

2. Chemical insults from environment, drugs, medications etc.

3. Emotional insults are the most complicated ones.

Emotional insults, are not well understood can be due to disappointment, failure, tragic event, fear and even bad dreams. (These insults do not apply to the people who commit crimes or wrong actions by pre-planning. Such pre-planned crimes or wrong actions aught to be due to bad mind. Such actions are criminal must have punishment).

Due to any types of insults/assaults, some neurons get affected and cease their normal function, leading to a shadow or a clouded mind. The clouded mind or the shadow is termed as a psychological condition or schizophrenia and other mental illness by the modern society. During such psychological impact, affected neurons cease the normal functional production of neurotrophins. The neurological insults may be manifested into jealousy, grief, greed and anger, in some cases violent crimes. Some of these manifestations may be reverted by taking a hot water bath, exercise, alcoholic drink or some kind of entertainment for diversion. However, in some cases it can become worse because the affected neurons become non functional and die off. Currently, there is no diagnostic test or specific treatment for mental illness including Schizophrenic psychosis and such prolonged condition is termed as depression..

Normal adults loose 0.2 % brain volume per year, whereas in patients with Alzheimer's disease the loss is greater. This is a clear indication that the death of neurons causing decrease level of neurotrophins may be manifesting the AD condition. As we age the population of neurons goes down decreasing the neurotrophin concentration. Thus, theoretically AD and aging can be controlled by neurotrophin treatment. However, neurotrophins having large in size blood-brain-barrier (BBB) is an obstacle. Small peptides having neurotrophic property is the best bate. Scientists are working towards finding such small molecules. Neurotrophic factors can not cross BBB due to their large size and therefore, cannot reach the brain when administered either orally or by injection.

Blood-Brain Barrier (BBB): Unlike all other organs BBB regulates substances entering the brain via the blood circulation system. This barrier is a unique defense system, which shuts out most toxins, bacteria and viruses which may be circulating in the blood, but allows the entry of necessary blood born molecules such as oxygen and glucose. The brain accounts for about 20 percent of the total oxygen consumption of the body, the energy associated with oxygen consumption comes from the utilization of glucose. Numerous chemical substances pass from the blood stream into the brain at rates that are far slower than for entry into all other organs in the body. Substances that find it difficult to get into the brain also find it exceedingly difficult to leave. The quality of BBB represented mainly by endothelial light junctions (LT) is now believed to be dependent and influenced by basal lamina of the micro vessels.

The high concentration of lipids is a unique feature of brain since about 50 percent of the dry weight of brain is lipid compared with 6 to 10 percent in other organs of the body. Although the function of the complex lipids is unknown, their implication in certain genetic types of mental retardation known as cerebral lipidoses is well documented. For example, in <u>Tay-Sachs</u> disease there is an accumulation of gangliosides, in <u>Gaucher disease</u> there is a rise in the cerebroside content of the brain, and in <u>Niemann-Pick</u> disease there is an accumulation of both sphingomyelin and gangliosides. It is also known that in demyelinating diseases the cerebroside and sphingomyelin content of the brain declines and there is a formation of cholesterol esters.

Three essential amino acids phenylalanine, tryptophan and histidine are associated with congenital errors of metabolism that produce mental retardation and they rise to neuroactive amines. Although the present evidence is not overwhelming, gamma-aminobutyric acid (GABA) has been implicated, both directly and indirectly, in the pathogenesis of Huntington's disease, Parkinsonism, epilepsy, Schizophrenia, tardive dyskinesias and senile dementia as well as several other behavioral disorders. GABA does not easily penetrate the BBB it is difficult to increase the brain concentrations of it by peripheral administration.

The endothelial cells of brain capillaries differ from those of other tissue such as muscle and heart in that the intercellular zones of membrane apposition are much more highly developed in the brain and are virtually continuous along all surface of these cells. Furthermore, cerebral vascular endothelial cells show a distinct lack of pinocytotic vesicles, which have been related to transvascular carrier systems of both large and small molecules. In a single individual organism, all of the somatic cells including the cells of the central and peripheral nervous system, possess entirely the same basic set of genetic information, with an exception of antibody producing lymphocytes.

Brief History of Psychology: Hippocrates (460-377 B.C.) a Greek physician who believed that mental disease was the result of natural causes of brain pathology rather than demonology. Galen (A.D. 130-200) believed that psychological disorders could have either physical causes, such as injuries to the head, or mental causes, such as disappointment in love. Martin Luther (1483-1546) the German theologian and the leader of the Reformation who held the belief, common to his time, that the mentally disturbed were possessed by the devil. Saint Teresa of Avila (1515-1582) a canonized Spanish nun who argued that mental disorder was an illness of the mind.

Dorothea Dix (1802-1887) an American teacher who founded the mental hygiene in the United States, which focused on the physical well-being of mental patients in hospitals. Franz Anton Mesmer (1734-1815) an Austrian physician who conducted early investigations into hypnosis as a medical treatment. Sigmund Freud (1856-1938) the founder of the school of psychological therapy known as psychoanalysis. William Healy (1869-1963) an American psychologist who established the Chicago Juvenile Psychopathic Institute and advanced the idea that mental illness was due to the environmental or socio cultural factors.

Treatments for Mental Illness: Genius is rarely if ever addressed in textbook of abnormal psychology, mental retardation almost always is. Nearly all of what we regard as "abnormal" in behavior we also regard as undesirable. As the notion spread in the Middle Ages that madness was caused by satanic possession, exorcism became a treatment of choice.

The mental institutes, once thought to be the most humane way to manage problems of the severely mentally ill, has now come to be seen as absolute or as an evil alternatives and is reviewed as more of a problem than a solution to the mental health. For centuries physicians sought a medicinal cure for mental disorders. One of the earliest extant treaties on the use of drugs to treat mental disorders is the work of Roman physician Galen, who coined the term apotherapy for the use of medications to treat human mental disorders. Most of his medications were laxatives and purgatives to clean the human body from materials believed to be causing the person's ills.

The Indian name in Hindi language for the root, "pagla-kadawa" means insanity herb. In 1931 Sen and Bose published an article in the Indian Medical journal about the usefulness of Rauwolfia in treating high blood pressure and insanity. In 1943 an article in the Indian Medical Gazette reported on the possible beneficial effects of the root for treating manic depression and schizophrenia. In 1950s the active ingredient in Rauwolfia, reserpine was isolated by Ciba, a Swiss drug company, (now it is Novartis). Today reserine has been surpassed as treatment of psychose because of the development of other drugs. The second psychoactive drug to emerge was chlorpromazine as a treatment for sever mental disorders.

There are more than one hundred drugs for the treatment of psychological illness. To name a few; Ambien, Ativan, Buspar and the most popular Prozac. Unfortunately, none of these drugs cure mental illness. On the contrary they show lot of intolerable side effects, some times even fatal. These drugs have complex effects, need different lengths of time to become effective and can influence different sorts of mental states in different ways. However, their efficacy can be compared to placebo effect. Studies on several drugs, such as dopamine, serotonine for treatment of mental illness in humans have yielded non conclusive results. Clinical trials with antidepressant drug MK-869 developed by Merck showed efficacy less than the placebo. Developing animal models for psychiatric disturbances is extremely difficult therefore, research for mental illness in animals is lacking.

Most of these drugs for treatment for mental illness have side effects which can range from minor to debilitating to even fatal. For example, the class of antidepressant, the monoamine oxidase inhibitors (MAOIs), can induce life threatening hypertension if the patient consumes any of various foods or other medicines on a warning list that includes cheese and cough syrup. Antipsychotic drug clozapine, can sometimes cause a deadly blood disorder called agranulocytosis. Anotherexample is the Thorazine that block the D_2 dopamine receptor can produce a Parkinsoniun syndrome called tardive dyskinesia.

Nerve growth factor (NGF) is required for the regulation, maintenance and survival of the neurons. Normal people loose 0.2% brain volume per year where as in AD the decrease is greater. As we grow older the neuron population goes down. Positive clinical effects have been reported after intracranial infusion of NGF to the single AD patient (Seiger et al. 1993). However, subsequent study with three more patients proved to be negative (Eriksdotter 1998).

The collaboration with Dr. Ericsson, M. D. Neurologist we performed pilot study of ten Alzheimer and ten Parkinson patients. In this study 750 µg of venom derived NGF was administered by nasal insufflations for a period of four weeks. The results were dramatic. The treated patients showed tremendous improvements in all usual symptoms. Although, NGF given by non invasive route was effective, continuous treatment could not be possible to get FDA approval, especially coming from snake venom.

It is imperative to discover small molecules having neurotrophic activity which can overcome blood-brain barrier. There are reports regarding the synthetic NGF peptide derivatives which prevent neuronal death and produce neurite outgrowth on rat adrenal pheochromocytoma (PC12) cells, the characteristic of neurotrophic factor (LeSautur et al. 1995). It was reported that the peptides corresponding to beta loop region of NGF were found to have the highest activity corresponding a loop 29-35 which is capable to interact with p75 receptor (Longo et al. 1933, 1997). AIT-082 is the first compound made by the company Neotherapeutics that entered human clinical trials for neuro-degenerative diseases, by oral administration. However, its efficacy was found to be marginal, showing no difference between Alzheimer's diseases patients treated with AIT-082 and placebo. As a result the company is out of business.

At Ophidia Products, Inc. we have identified the active domain for the biological activity of cobra venom derived NGF. The active domain consisting of ten amino acids, in its natural form or in synthetic version mimics the biological properties of the whole molecule NGF consisting of 116 amino acids. The synthetic version of the active domain is named ADESH which mimics the biological properties NGF in vitro and in vivo systems. ADESH can be made in abundance, and being a small molecule overcomes the blood-brain barrier. It can be administered by injection or can be taken by orally under the tongue.

Chapter 7
IN VIVO ANIMAL EXPERIMENTS

One year old Balb/c male mice are considered to be retired and non productive, were given ADESH orally for seven consecutive days and the controls received Phosphate buffer saline. Two days after the completion of the treatment the mice were sacrificed for organs. The organ homogenates were assayed for the NGF levels by ELISA (Lipps 2001, 2002). The results are presented graphically in figure 1.

Preparation of organ homogenates: One-year-old Balb/c male mice are considered as retired non productive were divided into two groups each consisting of five. Mice in group I were given orally 100 µg/mouse in 50 µl volume of ADESH, synthetic analog of NGF for seven consecutive days. The group II mice were given similar volume of PBS. Two days after the completion of the treatment the mice were sacrificed for organs. Organs from five of each group of mice were collected and one type of organs from five were pooled. The pool of the organs was homogenized in PBS by manual homogenizer. The homogenates were centrifuged and the supernatants for each pool organ were separated. Protein concentration for each supernatant was measured on spectrophotometer using a protein kit from Bio-Rad (USA catalogue 500-0006). The protein concentrations of the supernatants were adjusted to 100 µg/ml with PBS, as stocks for further testing.

Enzyme-Linked Immunosorbent Assay (ELISA): The binding

affinity of anti-ADSEH consisting of ten amino acids designated as AD-10, to various specimens known to contain NGF, such as body fluids, saliva, serum, urine etc. was studied by ELISA. The ELISA binding of anti-AD-10 was compared to anti-NGF from cobra venom. The tests were performed in 96 well micro titer plate. The wells of the plate were coated with one concentration of antigen (10 g/ml), diluted in carbonate-bicarbonate buffer pH 9.4 and each well received 100 µl. The plate was incubated at room temperature (RT) for 16 to 18 hours after which it was washed three times (3X) with PBS. The wells of the plate were blocked with 0.25ml/well of 3% Teleostean gelatin from cold water fish (Sigma) for 1/2 hour at RT. Anti-AD-10 and anti-NGFs, against V-NGF and H-NGF were diluted threefold in gelatin were added to the appropriate wells of ELISA plate, including positive and negative controls. The plate was incubated at 37°C for 1 to 1.5 hours. After washing 3X times horseradish peroxidase conjugated with IgG made in goat (Sigma) was added and incubated for 1 hour. Finally, the plate was washed and reacted with O-Phenylenediamine Dihydrochloride (OPD) for color development. The test was after 1/2 hour for ELISA titers.

Fig.1 . NGF concentration in organs of male mice before and after ADESH treatment.

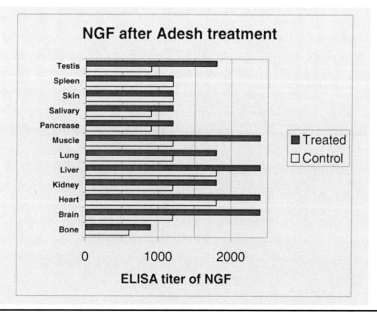

Fig. 1. It was revealed that there was increased in level of NGF in all organs of mice treated with ADESH in comparison to the controls. Most increased in NGF level was observed in brain, muscle and testis. These organs are most affected in old age. ADESH being a small molecule was able to pass through the BBB, reaching to the central nervous system; thereby exciting the neurons to produce more NGF in organs of the mice.

ADESH crosses Blood-Brain-Barrier:

Six months old Balb/c male mice were divided into three groups, each consisting of five and were treated orally for seven consecutive days as follows: Group I control mice were given PBS; Group II were treated with NGF 25 µg/mouse and the mice in Group III were treated with ADESH 100 µg/mouse. The mice were sacrificed for organs at 10 day Organ homogenates were assayed for NGF content by simple ELISA, using anti-NGF. figure 2.

Figure 2. ELISA titer /100 µl of NGF in organs of mice treated with NGF or ADESH in comparison to the controls.

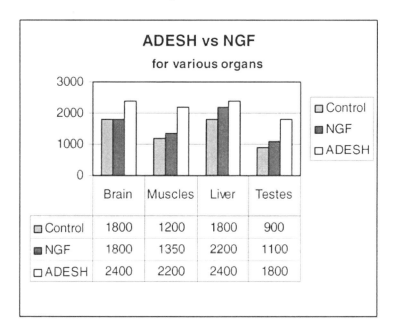

Results showed that there was no difference in NGF levels in brains of control and mice treated with NGF. NGF level in brain of mice treated with ADESH showed much higher levels of NGF than the respective controls. This shows that NGF did not pass through the BBB, unable to reach the brain to excite the neurons of the central nervous system (CNS) to make more NGF. On the other hand ADESH being a small molecule passed through BBB, reached CNS excited to produce more NGF. The homogenates of muscles, liver and testis showed little increase in NGF levels with NGF treatment acting on the peripheral nervous system (PNS) in comparison to the controls. However, there was reasonable increase in NGF in these organs with ADESH treatment. This proved that ADESH crosses BBB. This property is most essential for the treatment of neurological disorders.

From the literature it is clear that endogenously present protein NGF plays a role in displaying different disorders. Increased level of NGF is reported in patients with autoimmune disorders. My research reported the elevated level of NGF of patients suffering from allergy/asthma, diabetes mellitus, depression and various autoimmune disorders. To the contrary, my research has revealed that AD, PD and DS patients show low level of NGF. When we talk about elevated level for any protein in body fluids such as saliva, serum and urine means the loss of that protein from the organs. Therefore, decreased level of NGF manifests physical disorders like AD and PD and may be mental illness.

Chapter 8
TREATMENT FOR LOWERING IgE

IMMUNOGLOBULIN E (IgE) Elevated Level of IgE is a Culprit:

Asthma has increased dramatically worldwide over the past decades, particularly in developing countries and the experts are puzzling over the cause. Most asthma sufferers also have allergies. Not all people with allergies have asthma. Allergy is caused by variety of substances. Such substances stimulate, produce and release a group of antibodies known as immunoglobulin E (IgE). People with allergy and asthma appear to have a genetic predisposition for over producing IgE. During an allergic attack, these IgE antibodies can bind to special cells, called mast cells (MC), in the system, which are generally concentrated in the lungs, skin, and mucous membranes. Recent evidence is emerging that allergy can effect retina of eyes and lower the vision. This response triggers the release of number of active chemicals, responsible for over producing mucosa.

Human immunoglobulins are different types, such as IgG, IgA, IgM, IgD and IgE. IgG, IgA and IgM are protective immunoglobulins and the role of IgD may be implicated for food allergy. IgE is a minor component of the total immunoglobulin and is implicated in allergy, which in some cases manifests asthma. The presence of IgE in human serum was discovered in 1972 by Ishizaka and

Ishizaka. Allergic diseases are caused by adverse immune response to allergens. Allergens sensitized patients produce high levels of IgE, which manifest vasodilation, increased vascular permeability, edema, smooth muscle contraction and mucus secretion, resulting allergic reactions Ishizaka and Ishizaka (1984). Normal adults have 0.2 to 1.0 mg% of IgE. Currently, large percentage of the US population show higher than the normal range of allergy and the percentage is increasing every year.

IgE is implicated in asthma because asthma people show elevated levels of IgE. The level of total IgE in serum tends to correlate with disease severity, especially in respiratory allergies, Burrows et al. (1989), Sears et al. (1991). Allergic reaction causes inflammation and edema accumulating mast cells (MC) at the sites, which remain active for producing IgE under different conditions. Exercise and emotional stress activate MC to produce IgE induced allergy. Exercise induced asthma has been reported. This establishes the inter relationship between asthma and allergy.

Currently, IgE is assayed by radioimmunoassay (RIA), radio allergen absorbent test (RAST) or double sandwich ELISA, using blood serum or blood plasma. Few years ago I published a paper," Isolation of Nerve Growth Factor (NGF) from saliva, serum and urine" Because if this publication was invited to participate in the 6th Symposium on saliva at Egmond aan Zee, the Netherlands in 2002. I have developed a simple ELISA by using saliva. This is a first investigation reporting the use of non invasively collected saliva to assay IgE. Such simple ELISA test cannot be performed to assay any protein from serum or serum plasma. The test can be used to assay proteins present in serum, by using saliva. Whatever is present in serum is present in body fluids particularly saliva but in lesser concentration.

In this communication simple ELISA test comprising for example, an antigen NGF of saliva reacting with various concentrations of anti-NGF yielding ELISA titer/100 µl, at the lowest concentration of antibody. The endogenously present proteins, NGF, myoglobin, insulin and most importantly immunoglobulin IgE can be assayed by simple ELISA tests.

I always wonder about the therapeutics which worked in the past for mental illness quit working now. I am convinced by my research that this is due the elevated levels of IgE. We all have IgE, it is the elevated level excess of IgE interferes with the chemical drugs. IgE is a minor component of the total immunoglobulin and is implicated in allergy, which in some cases manifests asthma. Normal adults have 0.2 to 1.0 mg% of IgE. Currently, 60 % of the US population show higher than the normal range of IgE and the percentage is increasing every year. My research has shown that people suffering from allergy/asthma, diabetics, autoimmune diseases and depression show elevated level of IgE.

It is surprising to know that chemotherapy to some cancer patients produces side effects such as hair loss, skin rash, diarrhea etc while in others same drugs do not show any side effects. This may due to the elevated levels of IgE, causing interference and resistance to drugs. My research has revealed that elevated level of IgE is implicated in various disorders: (**1**) Diabetes, (**2**) Autoimmune diseases, (**3**) Allergy/Asthma, (**4**) Depression (**5**) Adverse side effects to the chemotherapy in cancer patients. (**5**). Osteoporosis (**6**) Chronic pain (**7**) Chronic inflammation and recently affects eye vision.

My research has proved that the elevated level of IgE is a culprit in manifesting numerous disorders, including diabetes. Therefore, it is imperative to have treatment to lower IgE level. By bringing the IgE level to normal the symptoms for allergy, asthma and mental disorders will be reduced. IgE level fluctuates according to the environment, therefore, continuous treatment is advocated, because the mast cells persist for a long period of time.

FDA approved Xolair, Genentech Corporation humanized monoclonal anti-IgE antibody for treatment of asthma for people over twelve years of age neutralizes IgE. Mono anti-IgE neutralize the circulating IgE and lowers its concentration. Xolair mono anti-IgE is restricted to people above 12 years of age. Its production is expensive, therefore it is a expensive and must be given by injection.

LETHAL TOXIN NEUTRALIZING FACTOR (LTNF)

Lethal Toxin Neutralizing Factor isolated from opossum serum having molecular weight 63.0 kDa, is a potent antidote for animal, plant and bacterial toxins (**US patent 5,576, 297** 1996). The active domain of the natural LTNF was identified, isolated and sequenced. After drug discovery, a synthetic peptide consisting of ten amino acids was constructed, named LT-10 having sequence from the N-terminal: L K A M D P T P P L Synthetic LT-10 proved to be an antidote for toxins derived from animal, plants-ricin and bacteria similar to natural LTNF, from opossum serum (**US Patent 5,744,449** 1998)

Although, LTNF was effective as a therapeutic we realized that the natural products for human use, coming from opossum serum will have dependence on the source and would require large number of opossums. Furthermore, LTNF is larger molecular weight protein is capable of of making antibodies and interfered the treatment. Therefore, it was imperative to make synthetic version of this amazing molecule for therapeutic purpose named LT-10 consisting of ten amino acids. The commonly held view that small synthetic peptides cannot mimic the effects of large polypeptide is by now considerably out of date (Wells,1996)[1]. Synthetic peptides can be produced cheaply in abundance. Furthermore, a peptide consisting of ten amino acids having low molecular weight can have better bio-availability.

CONVERSION OF ACTIVE DOMAIN OF NATURAL LTNF TO SYNTHETIC LT-10.

Lethal Toxin Neutralizing Factor (LTNF) was isolated from opossum serum having molecular weight 63 kDa is a potent antidote for toxins from animal, plant and bacteria. This part deals with the identification of a small fragment of LTNF eliciting the anti-lethal activity for animal plant and bacterial toxins, similar to natural LTNF. It was imperative to make synthetic version of this amazing molecule for therapeutic purpose.

Purified LTNF was treated with trypsin to cause fragmentation at the arginine and lysine sites. The fragments were separated by high pressure liquid chromatography (HPLC) and were tested versus anti-LTNF for binding affinity by enzyme-linked immunosorbent test (ELISA). The fragment showing the most binding to anti-LTNF was sequenced. Synthetic peptides consisting of 10 amino acids from the N-terminal were constructed and designated as LT-10, having amino acid sequence, Leu-Lys-Ala-Met-Asp-Pro-Thr-Pro-Pro-Leu.

Death due to intra muscular (IM) injection of predetermined lethal dose of toxins derived from animal, plant and bacteria in mice was prevented by the treatment of synthetic peptides LT-10. The lethality was inhibited when the treatment was given before or after the toxin injection. Synthetic LT-10 can be made in abundance and should become the universal therapy against intoxication caused by animal, plant and bacteria.

THERAPEUTIC APPLICATIONS OF LT-10

It is known that elevated level of immunoglobulin IgE is implicated in allergy/asthma. This research reports that the saliva of people suffering from diabetes II and various autoimmune diseases, including allergy asthma showed high level of IgE. The research also reports the use of non-invasively collected saliva for assaying IgE, and other endogenous proteins; nerve growth factor (NGF), myoglobin and insulin by simple ELISA test. Elevated IgE is a culprit for causing allergy/asthma, type II diabetes and autoimmune diseases. High level of IgE increases glucose concentration and disrupts the homeostasis of endogenous proteins.

LT-10 is a synthetic small peptide consisting of ten amino acids, the identified active domain of the lethal toxin neutralizing factor (LTNF). Both LTNF and LT-10 neutralize the lethality of animal, plant and bacterial toxins. Like toxins IgE is an allergen and therefore LT-10 must bind and neutralize it. This is a self case report where I was diagnosed for diabetes II based upon glucose level. I treated myself with LT-10 to lower IgE concentration, which brought the homeostasis of other endogenous proteins to normal state. Increased levels of these endogenous proteins manifests consequences e.g NGF for neuropathy, myoglobin for high blood pressure and insulin for diabetes II. LT-10 treatment reduced glucose and IgE levels bringing homeostasis of NGF, myoglobin and insulin to normal state. Therefore, LT-10 treatment is recommended for disorders implicated with high levels of IgE after FDA approval.

Saliva from normal people and patients suffering from type II diabetes, and various other disorders such as autoimmune diseases; were assayed for IgE, NGF, myoglobin and insulin by simple ELISA test using respective anti sera. It was revealed that the saliva specimens showed elevated levels of IgE, NGF, myoglobin and insulin in comparison to the controls from normal individuals.

IgE is a minor component of the total immune globulins of serum. Normal adults have 0.2 to 1.0 mg% of IgE. Allergic reactions caused by adverse immune response to allergen and IgE acts as an allergen. LT-10 binds to IgE similar way as to the toxins lowering the concentration of it. Thus LT-10 is a potent detoxicant for toxins and allergens. LT-10 acts like anti-IgE, it binds to IgE and lowers its concentration,

FDA approved Xolair, Genentech Corporation humanized monoclonal anti-IgE antibody for treatment of asthma for people over twelve years of age neutralizes IgE. LT-10 also neutralizes IgE. LT-10 has several advantages over mono anti-IgE. LT-10 is synthetic peptide made of ten amino acids, It can be made in abundance at low cost, where as the production of mono anti-IgE is expensive. LT-10 can be given under the tongue. Mono anti-IgE must be given by injection only. Both LT-10 and mono anti-IgE neutralize the circulating IgE and lowers its concentration. Percentage of asthma in children is increasing and mono anti-IgE is restricted to people above 12 years of age. For LT-10 there is no age limit.

Self Treatment Report: On my annual medical check, I was diagnosed to be diabetes based on the high level of glucose (142 mgs in the blood), the only available test for diagnosis. Glucose test is not reliable because it gives fluctuating readings. I did not have discomfort or any other symptoms. After two months of Glucotrol (Pfizer) treatment and sugar free diet, the blood glucose level came down to 120. I am allergic to insects bites, and therefore IgE level in my blood serum has been higher than the normal range. In 2000 I published a paper "Isolation of nerve growth factor (NGF) from human body fluids; saliva, serum and urine". Because of this publication I was invited to Netherlands in 2002 to make a presentation at the 6th European Symposium on saliva. Meantime, I discovered that IgE and other proteins, myoglobin and insulin can be assayed from saliva.

The following experiments were performed. Fasting saliva was collected and blood glucose level was measured for seven consecutive days for each experiment. Sugar free diet was observed for the entire period of experiments. Four days waiting period was allowed before starting the next experiment The saliva samples were collected for each experiment. Besides glucose, IgE, NGF, myoglobin and insulin were assayed in saliva.

Experiment # 1: No treatment
Experiment # 2: Glucotrol treatment, 10 mgs in the morning and 5 mgs in the evening.
Experiment # 3: LT-10 treatment, 2 mgs/day, 1 mg in the morning and 1 mg in the evening.
Experiment # 4: Combination of 15 mgs/day Glucotrol and LT-10, 2 mgs/day.

Followings observations can be made:

1. IgE levels remained high, unchanged in expts.#1 and #2 with no treatment or Glucotrol treatment respectively. This shows that Glucitrol treatment has no effect on lowering IgE, High level of glucose is considered as the cause of diabetes and Glucotrol treatment lowers it,

2. LT-10 treatment alone or in combination of Glucotrol lowered IgE levels in expts.#3 and #4, greater in expt.#3 than in expt.#4. This emphasizes that LT-10 alone lowers the IgE level and glucose concentration.

3. NGF levels remained high in expts.#1 and #2. LT-10 treatment alone or in combination of Glucotrol lowered NGF levels in expts.#3 and #4, greater in expt.#3 with LT-10 treatment alone than with the combination of LT-10 and Glucotrol.

4. Glucotrol alone as in expt.#2 or in combination with LT-10 as in expt.#4 increased the concentration of myoglobin. This may be the side effect of Glucotrol treatment. Increased myoglobin is implicated in causing high blood pressure, leading to heart attack.

5. Insulin levels decreased in expts.#2, #3 and #4. Glucotrol alone as expt.#2 and in combination with LT-10 lowered insulin levels as in expts 2 amd 4. The increased level of insulin in other words loss of it causes the manifestation of diabetes, therefore, insulin is given by injection to diabetes patients.

My research proves that the elevated level of IgE is a culprit in manifesting numerous disorders, including diabetes. The results of the above experiments proved that LT-10 treatment brings down the level of IgE. After bringing IgE level to normal status the NGF level comes to the normal state. High levels of proteins detected in body fluids means the loss of those from the system. Loss of NGF causes neuropathy, loss of myoglobin cause heart problems and insulin causes diabetes. It seems controlling IgE level will solve many health problems.

IgE level fluctuates according to the environment, therefore, continuous LT-10 treatment is advocated, because the mast cells persist for a long period of time. I have been treating myself with LT-10 for last several years to maintain the levels of IgE, NGF, myoglobin and insulin to normal state. LT-10 is non toxic. I strongly advocate after FDA approval LT-10 treatment for lowering IgE concentration, By lowering the IgE level the concentration of NGF, myoglpbin, insulin and may be other endogenous proteins, like cytokines can be restored.

High Level of IgE Causes Diaberes Type II

Diabetes is two types: Type I insulin dependent and type II, insulin independent referred as diabetes mellitus, is a syndrome which affects many systems. Diabetes mellitus is a common condition, occurs in high percentage of human population during middle age. Currently, the elevated glucose in the blood is the only criterion upon which diagnosis of diabetes mellitus is based, because there are no specific markers. It is believed that insufficiency of metabolically active insulin may be implicated in the development of long micro-vascular and neurological complications of diabetes. Recent research suggests the hypothesis that elements of the innate immune system, such as cytokines or the acute phase reactants that stimulate, contribute to the development of type II diabetes and obesity, Festa et al. (2000). The publication by Lindsey et al.(2001) states that elevated levels of gamma globulins in blood can predict type II diabetes in Pima Indian population.

There are publications stating that several inflammatory and autoimmune diseases are characterized by an altered concentration of circulating nerve growth factor (NGF). Levels of NGF in serum of patients with inflammatory autoimmune disorders such as chronic arthritis (CA); systemic sclerodermia (SS); systemic lupus erythematosus (SLE) and multiple sclerosis (MS) were compared with the normal controls. It was reported that MS patients showed the highest level of NGF and CA patients showed the lowest in comparison to normal controls. Also SLE and SS patients showed higher levels of NGF in comparison to normal controls Bracci-Laudiero et al. (1992, 1993); Aloe et al. (1994); Bonin et al. (1996). Emotional stress induced by parachute jumping changes blood nerve growth factor levels and the distribution of nerve growth factor receptors in lymphocytes, Aloe et al. (1994).

As early as 1961, Reid demonstrated that myoglobinuria is one of the characteristic symptoms in human snakebite victims, Reid (1961). The presence of myoglobin in serum and urine was reported as an early marker for kidney dysfunction, Wu et al. (1994).

From the above-cited literature it is clear that endogenous proteins such as IgE, NGF, myoglobin, and insulin play role in displaying different diseases/disorders. This investigation reports the elevated level of IgE in saliva of patients suffering from diabetes mellitus, causes disruption for other endogenous important proteins. The investigation reports that the homeostasis of the endogenous major proteins; NGF, myoglobin and insulin is disrupted due to elevated levels of IgE.

I tested saliva from five patients diagnosed for diabetes, versus normal people for IgE, NGF, myoglobin and insulin. These diabetic patients are under treatment for a long time.

Table 1. IgE Titer/100 µl in saliva of normal people compared to Type II diabetes patients

Controls normal	ELISA titer/100µl	Diabetes patients	ELISA titer/100µl
1	12150	1A	145800
2	12000	2A	145800
3	11550	3A	136000
4	12050	4A	150000
5	12500	5A	145800
Average	**12050**	Average	**144680**

Results of table 1 show that IgE titers are consistently higher in diabetes type II patients in comparison to the controls. The average

IgE level is **12 X** higher than in the controls, derived by average titer of diabetes divided by the average titer of controls 144680 divided by 12050 = 12. The elevated level of IgE is the main cause of diabetes showing rise in glucose level only diagnostic marker for diabetes.

Table 2. NGF titer/100 µl in saliva of normal people compared to type II diabetes patients

Controls normal	ELISA titer/100µl	Diabetes patients	ELISA titer/100µl
1	1200	1A	24300
2	1500	2A	5400
3	1250	3A	5450
4	1400	4A	21000
5	1200	5A	5400
Average	**1310**	Average	**12310**

Table 2 shows that NGF titers are consistently higher in diabetes type II patients in comparison to the controls. The average NGF level is **9.3 X** higher than in the controls, derived by average titer of diabetes divided by average titer of normal which is 9.3 times. The loss of NGF from the body causes neuropathy, inflammation and it is due to the elevated level of IgE.

Table 3. Myoglobin titer/100 µl in saliva of normal people compared to type II diabetes patients

Controls normal	ELISA titer/100µl	Diabetes patients	ELISA titer/100µl
1	1800	1A	3600
2	2700	2A	10800
3	1500	3A	5450
4	1850	4A	7200
5	2100	5A	5400
Average	**1990**	Average	**6480**

Results of table 3 show that myoglobin titers are consistently higher in diabetes type II patients in comparison to the controls.

The average myoglobin level in diabetes patients was **3.2 X** than in the controls, derived by average titer of diabetes divided by average titer of controls. It is reported and accepted that the increased level of myoglobin is prone to give high blood pressure leading to heart attacks.

Table 4. Insulin titer/100 µl in saliva of normal people compared to type II dibetes patients

Controls normal	ELISA titer/100µl	Diabetes patients	ELISA titer/100µl
1	450	1A	1800
2	600	2A	1800
3	M500	3A	2800
4	550	4A	2700
5	600	5A	2750
Average	**540**	Average	**2370**

Table 4 shows that insulin titers are consistently higher in diabetes type II patients in comparison to the controls. The average insulin level in diabetes patients is **4.3 X** than in the controls, derived by average titer of diabetes divided by average titer of controls. It is accepted that diabetic type II is due to loss of insulin from the system. Therefore, diabetic patients are treated with insulin or the insulin producing chemicals. Thus the elevated level of IgE is responsible for causing diabetes II

I received ten saliva specimens from Dr. Ericsson, M. D. Neurologist, of the patients with various types of auto immune diseases. I tested ten saliva specimens from normal people to compare with saliva from autoimmune patients for IgE, NGF, myoglobin and insulin. These patients are under treatment for a long time.

Table 5. ELISA titer/100 µl for IgE in saliva of normal people and patients with autoimmune disease

Controls normal	ELISA titer/100µl	Autoimmune patients	ELISA titer/100µl
1	12150	1A	145800
2	12000	2A	145800
3	11550	3A	138000
4	12050	4A	150000
5	12500	5A	145800
6	12300	6A	140000
7	11050	7A	139000
8	12000	8A	155000
9	12500	9A	144000
10	11550	10A	145500
Average	**11965**	**Average**	**144890**

Results of table 5 showed that IgE titers were consistently higher in autoimmune disease patients in comparison to the controls. The average IgE level was **12.1 X** than in the controls, derived by dividing the average titer of autoimmune disease, 144890 by average titer of controls 11965, equals to 12.1. This shows that IgE level is several times hiher than the normal people. It can be safely stated that autoimmune disease patients suffer from allergy.

Table 6. ELISA Titer/100 µl for NGF in saliva of normal people and patients with autoimmune disease

Controls normal	ELISA titer/100µl	Diabetes patients	ELISA titer/100µl
1	1200	1A	24300
2	1500	2A	5400
3	1250	3A	5450
4	1400	4A	21000
5	1200	5A	5450
6	1250	6A	24000
7	1300	7A	5500
8	1250	8A	5400
9	1450	9A	20000
10	1400	10A	5600
Average	**1320**	**Average**	**12210**

Table 6 showed that NGF titers were consistently higher in autoimmune disease patients in comparison to the controls. The average NGF level is **9.25 X** higher than in the controls, derived by average titer of autoimmune disease divided by average titer of the normal, which is 9.3.

Because the IgE is high it causes loss of NGF which is responsible for neuropathy and inflammation in autoimmune disease patients.. Therefore, patients with autoimmune disease feel tired short of stamina.

Table 7. ELISA Titer/100 µl for myoglobin in saliva of normal people and patients with autoimmune disease.

Controls normal	ELISA titer/100µl	Diabetes patients	ELISA titer/100µl
1	1800	1A	3600
2	2700	2A	10800
3	1500	3A	5450
4	1850	4A	7200
5	2100	5A	5400
6	2000	6A	8100
7	1850	7A	5400
8	1550	8A	7400
9	1600	9A	3600
10	1550	10A	3650
Average	**1850**	**Average**	**6060**

Results of table 7 showed that myoglobin titers were consistently higher in autoimmune disease patients in comparison to the controls. The average myoglobin level in autoimmune disease patients was **3.3 X** than in the controls, derived by average titer of autoimmune disease divided by average titer of controls. IgE increases the myoglobin which causes high blood pressure leading to heart attacks.

Table 8. ELISA Titer/100 µl for Insulin in saliva of normal people and patients with autoimmune disease

Controls normal	ELISA titer/100µl	Diabetes patients	ELISA titer/100µl
1	450	1A	1800
2	600	2A	1800
3	500	3A	2800
4	550	4A	2700
5	600	5A	2750
6	650	6A	1850
7	600	7A	1900
8	600	8A	2500
9	450	9A	2350
10	500	10A	2400
Average	**550**	**Average**	**2285**

Table 8 showed that insulin titers were consistently higher in autoimmune disease patients in comparison to the controls. The average insulin level in autoimmune patients was **4.15 X** than in the controls, derived by average titer of autoimmune disease divided by average titer of the controls. The loss of insulin from the system due to the elevated IgE may cause diabetes in some autoimmune patients.

Figure 3 shows the graphic presentation of IgE, NGF, myoglobin and insulin in normal people versus times the concentration in autoimmune patients. Normal people have IgE, NGF, myoglobin and insulin, therefore he value of IgE, NGF, myoglobin and insulin of normal people was considered as 1. Times concentration for IgE, NGF, myoglobin and insulin was derived by dividing the average ELISA titers of autoimmune disease patients by normal people.

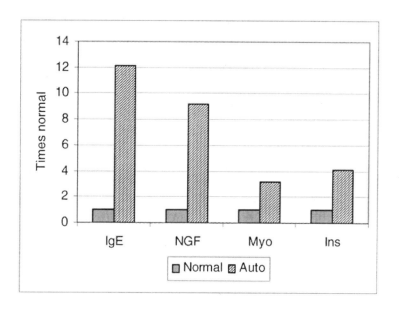

Figure 3 shows the graphic presentation of IgE, NGF, myoglobin and insulin in normal people versus times the concentration in autoimmune patients. The value of IgE, NGF, myoglobin and insulin of normal people was considered as 1. Times concentration for IgE, NGF, myoglobin and insulin was derived by dividing the average ELISA titers of autoimmune disease patients by normal people.

I collected saliva specimens from the patients suffering from various disorders, were assayed for IgE, NGF, Insulin and Myoglobin

Specimen	Status	IgE	NGF	Insulin	Myoglobin
Pool of 10	Normal	1.0	1.0	1.0	1.0
JC	Diabetes	12.0	20.5	4.0	6.0
TF	Asthma	12.0	4.5	6.0	3.0
WK	Depression	18.0	20.5	4.0	9.0
GK	Osteoporosis	6.0	2.25	2.0	1.5
RC	Arthritis	4.0	3.5	1.0	4.0

Table 9. Comparison of Concentration of IgE, NGF, Insulin and Myoglobin in patients with various disorders. Expressed as times X, considering the value 1 for normal

Results showed that the levels of IgE, NGF, Insulin and myoglobin are consistently higher in the saliva of patients suffering from various disorders such as asthma, depression, osteoporosis and arthritis, in comparison to the pool of ten normal individuals. The results shows emphatically that elevated level of IgE is a culprit responsible for the cause of these disorders.

Chapter 8
STRATEGY FOR TREATMENT OF MENTAL ILLESS

The era of Freud and the era of de institutionalization are ending. The era of neurobiology has begun and promises to revolutionize our understanding of the brain and its diseases. Neurobiology is a science of brain and psychology is science of mind. The authors of the book Out of its Mind chose to call new psychology "neurodynamics". The combination of neurobiology and psychology binds to neurodynamics, which is strictley related to the brain. Therefore, I have named my book **"Neurodynamics of Mind"** which covers both the brain and the mind.

LT-10 treatment is recommended: My research has revealed that high level of IgE is a culprit for causing resistant to the drugs used to work for the treatment of various disorders. Currently, in the US more than 60 % population show higher levels of IgE. Therefore, I advocate that all people should be screened for IgE levels. Individuals showing elevated levels of IgE, at least two to three times than the normal, should be treated with LT-10 to bring the level down. One mg % or less of IgE is considered normal.

The people suffering from different disorders, after bringing the IgE level to normal status the currently used drugs may be more effective. Conversely, bringing IgE level to normal, the concentration of other endogenous proteins such as NGF, myoglobin and insulin etc. will come to the normal status. Loss of NGF causes neuropathy, loss of myoglobin causes heart problems and insulin causes diabetes. It seems controlling IgE level will solve many health problems. In other words, there is a need for the treatment of allergy.

The elevation of IgE is implicated in many disorders for which the etiology or causative agents are not known. There are no diagnostic markers for these disorders. At least in case of diabetes glucose concentration is a accepted diagnostic test which is unreliable. It seems that we need a treatment for allergy and currently there is no specific treatment. My search revealed that the elevated level of IgE causes the increase in glucose. The currently used drugs for treating diabetes are those having ability to lower glucose, but they also produce side effects. I believe that **LT-10 is a great discovery after that of penicillin.** After FDA approval LT-10 treatment will improve the health and quality of millions of lives of people afflicted with various disorders.

IgE level fluctuates according to the environment. Therefore, LT-10 treatment should be continuous, because the mast cells persist for a long period of time. The people suffering from different disorders, after bringing the IgE level to normal status the currently used drugs may be more effective. Conversely, bringing IgE level to normal, concentration other endogenous proteins such as NGF, myoglobin and insulin etc. come to the normal status. Loss of NGF causes neuropathy, loss of myoglobin cause heart problems and insulin causes diabetes. It seems controlling IgE level will solve many health problems.

ADESH Treatment for Psychological Disorders and Arresting Aging : Normal adults loose 0.2 % brain volume per year. Different types of insults can cause a change in the concentration of neurotrophins and imbalanced in homeostatis, leading to schizophrenic psychosis and other mental illness. The insults can be physical trauma, chemicals, and emotional. Neurotrophic factor hypothesis states that developing neurons compete with each other for a limited supply of neurotrophic factor/s provided by the target tissue.

Successful competitors survive, unsuccessful ones die. Loss of neurotrophic factor/s may cause manifestation of Alzheimer's disease or schizophrenia. Therefore, treatment with ADESH can restore the affected neurons which are failing to perform their task. The loss of failing neurons can happen due to aging and insults.

Normal adults loose 0.2 % brain volume meaning number of neurons. If normal people are treated with ADESH they will not contract meurological or mental disorders. The continuous treatment with ADESEH will enable failing neurons to remain active and prevent from death. Thus, besides not contracting diseases their aging process will be arrested.

ADESH Treatment for Neurological Disorders: Normal adults loose 0.2 % brain volume per year where as in patients with Alzheimer's disease the loss is greater. My research has shown that people suffering from AD, PD and DS show low concentration of NGF in comparison to the normal individuals. These people should be treated with ADESH to activate the failing neurons to produce and increase the NGF concentration. My research showed that one year old male mice after treating with ADESH orally, increased the level of NGF in all organs and significantly more in brain, muscle and testis. These are the organs most affected in old age. ADESH activates the neurons of CNS and PNS enabling them to generate more NGF. ADESH is advocated for the treatment of:

1. Psychological Disorders; depression, paranoia, schizophrenia

2. Neurological Disorders, AD, PD, DS and other.

3. Arresting Aging, improving impotency.

DISCUSSION

LTNF a Universal Antitoxicant: Snakebite continues to be a major medical problem among rural communities of developing countries. The experimental preparation of anti-Naja serum by Calmette in 1894, led Vital Brazil (1898) to make the first polyvalent serum against *Bothrops jararaca* and *Crotalus durissus terrificus* for therapeutic use. Since then, equine antivenoms are in practice for the treatment of snakebites, although side effects associated with the sensitivity to equine protein occur in about 70% of all treatments. Apparently, the risk of death from serious snakebite poisoning is greater than the risk of side effects of the anti venom therapy.

Non-equine anti venom would be a comfort to those especially sensitive to horse proteins. Few years ago, UK based Therapeutic Antibodies Inc. produced anti venom in sheep to overcome the horse protein allergy problem. However, 20% of the treated patients in clinical trials showed serum sickness to sheep anti venom also. The company went out of business.

For many years, Wyeth-Ayerst was the sole producer of anti venom made in horses, for the treatment of snakebites in North and Central America. For world wide anti venoms are made against the venoms of snakes prevalent to the region. As a result there are numerous anti venoms made by more than 70 different producers. Wyeth anti venoms are made against the venoms of species of snakes, prevalent to North and Central America and those are, *C. atrox, C. durrisus terrificus* and *Agkistrodon bothrops*. Thus, Wyeth's anti venom is effective only for the snakebites of these species. On the other hand, LT-10 is effective against the venoms of all species of snakes. Therefore, LT-10 can become a universal treatment for snakebites. Furthermore, LT-10 is effective against scorpion and bee venoms, plant derived ricin and botulinum toxin. Therefore, LT-10 can become an universal treatment for toxins derived from animals, plants and bacteria. In the standard treatment for snakebite massive amounts of anti venom is administered for effectiveness, even though a large percentage of the population is hypersensitive to anti venom made in horses. Under such conditions LT-10 should be a most favorable replacement. It is further anticipated that the LT-10 invention has military applications due to the variety of unknown exposures that can occur under military conditions.

LT-10 Treatment for IgE Implicated Disorders: Human immunoglobulins are different types, such as IgG, IgA, IgM, IgD and IgE. IgG, IgA, IgM are protective immunoglobulins. IgE is a minor component of the total immunoglobulins and it is implicated in allergy, which in some cases manifests asthma. Normal adults have 0.2 to 1.0 mg% of IgE. IgE is considered to be like allergen. Allergic diseases are caused by adverse immune response to allergens. IgE is implicated in asthma because asthma patients show high levels of IgE. My research has revealed that high level of IgE is implicated in: **1.** Type II diabetes; **2.** Various types of Autoimmune diseases; **3.** Depression; **4.** Asthma; **5.** Chronic wounds and burns; and **6.** adverse side effects and resistance to cancer therapy.

It was revealed that the level of IgE in patients of these disorders is several times higher than the control normal individuals. It was further revealed that **A.** patients showing elevated level of IgE, showed higher concentration of myoglobin, may become prone to have high blood pressure. **B.** Patients having high level of IgE, showed elevated glucose, are diagnosed as diabetes. **C.** Patients of autoimmune disease showed high level of nerve growth factor (NGF), which may be causing neuropathy and inflammation. The patients suffering from allergy/asthma, diabetes, autoimmune diseases, chronic wounds and burns are under standard treatments for years for their respective cause. We believe that overall elevated levels of IgE may be interfering and resisting the treatment. Therefore, it is imperative that IgE levels should be brought down. By bringing IgE level to normal state the treatment will become more effective.

Genentech Corp. has proposed monoclonal antibody (Mono anti-IgE) as a treatment for asthma. Administration of monoclonal antibody is a passive process of immunization. The life period of such passive antibody is limited. Furthermore, the unutilized Mono anti-IgE is liable to generate anti-anti-IgE or anti-idiotypic antibody, which is a copy of IgE, will cause interference. Elevated levels of IgE are implicated in several disorders. The proposed treatment with LT-10 lowers the concentration of IgE (**PCT /US03/01044** issued in 2003). LT-10 has several advantages over Mono anti-IgE. LT-10 is a synthetic peptide made of 10 amino acids, which can be made in abundance and at low cost, whereas Mono anti-IgE is a large protein molecule and expensive. LT-10 can be given orally under the tongue. Mono anti-IgE must be given by injection only. Both LT-10 and Mono anti-IgE neutralize the circulating IgE and lower the IgE level. The percentage of asthma in children is increasing, but Mono anti-IgE is restricted to people above 12 years of age. However, for LT-10 there is no age limit. Excess LT-10 in the system will not do any harm. Excess of Mono anti-IgE unused will make antibodies. These anti idiotypic antibodies, or anti-anti-Mono IgE, which is a copy of IgE, will interfere with treatment.

We propose continuous treatment with LT-10e in order to maintain normal IgE level. Mast cells persist for a long period of time and secrete IgE under environmental conditions, emotional stress, or exercise, etc. On the other hand, Mono anti-IgE treatment cannot be given continuously due to the route and expense, etc.

Currently, diabetes, depression and autoimmune diseases are treated with various drugs. LT-10 treatment lowers the IgE level and encourages the homeostasis of other proteins, which improves the symptoms in people afflicted with these diseases. We believe that non-toxic LT-10 treatment is ideal and it is waiting for FDA approval.

REFERENCES

Adler L., Pachtman E., Franks R., Pecevich M., Waldo M. and Freedman R. (1982). Neurological evidence for defect in neuronal mechanisms involved in sensory gating in schizophrenia. Biol,. Psychiatry **17:** 639-654.

Adler L., Rose G. and Freedman R. (1986). Neurological studies of sensory gating in rats, effects of amphetamine, phenycyclidine and mhaloperiol. Biol,. Psychiatry 21, 787-798n.

Akabarian D., Vinuela A., Kim J. J., Potkin S. G., Bunney W. E. and Jones E. G. (1993). Distorted distribution of nicotinamide-adenine dinucleotide phosphatase neurons lobe of schizophrenics implies anomalous cortical development. Arch. Gen. Psychiatry 50, 178-187.

Aloe, Bracci-Laudiero L, Alleva E. etal. (1994). Emotional stress induced by parachute junping changes blood nerve growth factor levels and the distribution of nerve growth factor receptors in lymphocytes. Proc. Natl. Acad. Sci. USA 91:10440-10444.

Anderson M. C., Ochsner K. N., Kuhl B. et al.(2004). Neural systems underlying the suppression of unwanted memories. Science 303:232-235

Barde Y. A. (1989) Trophic factors and neuronal survival. Neuron 2: 1525-1534.

Benes F. M. (1989). Myelination of cortical-hipocampal relays during late adolescence. Schizophre. Bull. 15, 585-593.

Benes F. M., Sorenson I. and Bird E.D. (1991). Reduced neuronal size in posterior hippocampus of schizophrenic patients. Schizophre. Bull.17, 597-608.

Benes F. M., Sorenson I. Vincent S. L., Bird E.D. and Sathi M. (1992). Increased density of glutamate-immunoreactive vertical processes in superficial laminae on cingulated cortex of schizophrenic brain. Cerebral Cortex 2, 503-512.

Berger P. A., and Barchas J. D. (1983). Pharmacolgic studies of beta-endorphin in psychopathology. Psychiatr. Clin. North Am. 6, 377-391.

Cohen, S. (1959) Purification and metabolic effects of nerve growth promoting protein from snake venom. J. Biol. Chem 234: 1129-1137.

Crome L. Stern J. (1972) Pathology of mental retardation, 2nd Edition, Churchill Livingstone.

Davis T. P. Culling-Berglund A. J. and Schoemaker H. (1986). Specific regional differences of in vitro beta-endorphin metabolism metabolism in schizophrenics. Life Sci. 39, 2601-2609.

Delabar j. M. et al. (1987). Beta amyloid gene triplication in Alzheimer's disease and karyotypically normal Down syndrome. Science 235:1300-1392.

Eisenberger, N. I., Liberman, M. D. and Williams, K. D. (2003). Does rejection hurt? An FMRI study of social exclusion. 302: 290-292.

Fayer J. (1869) Death from snakebites: a trial condensed from the sessions report. Ind. Med. Gaz. 4, 156.

Hefti F. (1983) Alzheimer;s disease caused by a lack of nerve growth factor. Ann. Neurol. 13:109-110.

Hefti F., Weiner W. J. (1986) Nerve growth factor and Alzheimer's disease. Ann. Neurol. 20:275-281.

LeSauter L. et al. (1995). Small peptide mimetics of nerve growth factor bund TrKA receptors and effects biological responses. J. Biol. Chem 270:6564-6569.

Levi-Montalcini R, Myer H, Hamburger V. (1954) In vitro experiments on the effects of mouse sarcoma on spinal and sympathetic ganglia of chick embryo. Cancer Res.14: 49-57.

Lipps B. V. (1998). Biological and immunological properties of nerve growth factor from snake venoms. Journal of Natural Toxins, 7:121-130.

Lipps B. V. (2000). Detection of nerve growth factor (NGF) in venoms from diverse source: Isolation and characterization of NGF from the venom of honeybee (*Apis melifera*). Journal of Natural Toxins, 9:13-19.

Lipps B. V. (2000). Isolation of nerve growth factor (NGF) from human body fluids; saliva, serum and urine: Comparison between cobra venom and cobra serum NGF. Journal of Natural Toxins, 9:349-356.

Lipps B. V. (2001). Isolation and characterization of nerve growth Factor (NGF) excreted from cultured eukaryotic cells. Journal of Natural Toxins, 10:213-219.

Lipps B. V. (2001). Decreased levels of nerve growth factor in organs of mice as a consequence of sub-lethal Injection of cobra venom. Journal of Natural Toxins, 10: 283-290.

Lipps B. V. (2002). Restoration of nerve growth factor in organs of mice injected with cobra venom followed by specific treatment and reversal period. Journal of Natural Toxins, 11, 87-93.

Lipps B. V. (2002). Assay of specific antibodies produced in organs of mice immunized with nerve growth factor. Journal of Natural Toxins 11: 149-153.

Lipps B. V. (2002). Age and sex-related difference in levels of nerve growth factor in organs of BALB/c mice. Journal of Natural Toxins 11: 387-391.

Longo F. M. et al. (1997). Synthetic NGF peptide derivatives present neuronal death via a p75 receptor dependant mechanism. J. Neuroscience Res. 48:1-17.

Mann D. M., Yates P. O. (1984) Alzheimer's presenile dementia, senile dementia of Alzheimer type and down syndrome in middle age. Applied Neurobiol. 10: 185-207.

Mckinney W. and bunney W. (1969) Animal models of depression. 1. review of evidence, implications for research. Arch. Psychiatry 21, 240-248.

Phelps C. et al. (1989) Potential use of nerve growth factor to treat Alzheimer's disease. Neurobiol. Aging 10:205-207.

Thome J. Johnson E. et al. (1997) Ciliary neurotrophic factor null mutation and schizophrenic in Swedish population. Psychiatr. Geret. 7:79-82.

Thome J. Foley P. Riederer P. (1998). Neurotrophic factors and the maldevelmental hypothesis of schizophrenic psychoses. Review article. J. Neur. Trasm. 105:85-100.

Stephan, K. E. and Marshall, J. C. (2003). Lateralized cognitive processes and lateralized task control in human brain, Science 301: 384-389.

Yuen E. C., Mobley W. C. (1996). Therapeutic potential of neurotrophic factors for neurological disorders. Ann. Neurol. 40:346-354.